WE CAN BREATHE AGAIN

THE DISCOVERY OF A NATURAL THERAPY FOR ASTHMA

WE CAN BREATHE AGAIN

THE DISCOVERY OF A NATURAL THERAPY FOR ASTHMA

Dr Machi Mannu

Published by MedB
www.medb.es

Cover Photo and Illustration Erkaim Baisheva

Edited by Philip and Violet King

First edition 2017

Printed by CreateSpace

ISBN: 978-0-9957757-1-8

Dedication

For Mum who thankfully kept me alive with the help of chemical drugs, and for my Nan who inspired me to find another way.

CONTENTS

Introduction 1

The Problem with the Current Medical
Management of Asthma 7

The Discovery of NGC Therapy 15

Environmental and Health Factors Affecting
Asthma..47

References..67

About the Author..79

Introduction

Lying on a trolley in the emergency room surrounded by people and medical equipment, I remember thinking how slow they were to respond to my situation. No one seemed to be acting in the way I was trained to respond to asthma emergencies. To quickly secure a line for life-saving intravenous hydrocortisone, aminophylline, etc., drugs I had administered countless times to people in my situation.

I wondered "how I had allowed my health to deteriorate to such a state?" Those were my last thoughts before I lost consciousness and spent the next five days in a coma.

My earliest memories are of my asthma attacks. Asthma runs in my family, affecting only the males. My Father, Brothers and Cousins all have asthma or respiratory problems to varying degrees. I suffered severe and chronic asthma in childhood. My Mum, an expert nurse, kept me alive during those most difficult periods of my life. Many a night I would wake up to her administering an intravenous drug to relieve the severe midnight attacks I was prone to having.

I used inhalers all the time as a child, and those times when inhalers failed to provide sufficient relief, my Mum would take over with intravenous medications. Even then, there were periods when every form of therapy failed, including weeks of hospital admission. In those desperate times my Nan, my Dad's Mum would be invited into the picture. She always worked her magic. A herbalist and midwife, she would come with her potions which I would drink, eat or inhale under her wrapper.

Her therapy always worked when others have failed, and as I grew older, I took only her therapy. I believe that the last four years of my teenage years when I was free from asthma was a result of her treatment. My regret is that she passed on before I had sense enough to appreciate and learn her techniques.

Later, the asthma attacks came back, but I was already in medical school and had thoroughly learned everything I could about managing asthma.

So right up until I suffered the coma, I never imagined I could end up in an emergency from asthma. It could happen to people I treated, but surely not to me!

Nevertheless, there were clear signs in the months preceding the coma that my health was spiralling downwards. As an adult, the attacks I suffered were never of the same severity as in my childhood, but in the months leading up to the coma, the relatively minor asthma attacks I occasionally suffered became more intense. I started taking more medications and was also suffering from other health problems - fatigue, joint pains, stomach problems and irregular heartbeats. I was alarmed by my failing health and even more concerned that the drugs that I had grown to rely on were now failing me.

My childhood healing experience with my Nan encouraged me to take a critical look at natural therapies. I set up a health clinic, MedB Diagnostics, and with the aid of an advanced diagnostic and analytic technology, I started researching and using natural products, selecting only products that had a long history of use and backed by scientific studies. My research had been going on for a couple of months before I had the coma.

After my experience in the hospital which was both terrifying and traumatic, I died for five days; I channelled my energy into finding a natural remedy for asthma. I was the perfect guinea pig, and I tried out everything natural that I could find that is believed to help with asthma. I tried corrective breathing techniques, salt inhalation, and urine therapy. I tried dozens of supplements, herbs and potions. Nothing made any difference. I was not searching for a cure; rather I was searching for a natural medication that would produce a quick and noticeable relief from asthma symptoms.

It took a while, but eventually, I came upon what I thought 'could' be the remedy that I had been searching for. The relief I experienced when I first tried it encouraged me, and in the last four years, I have developed and tested an effective variation of that remedy.

Since discovering the treatment which I call the NGC therapy, my health has improved immensely. All the other health problems I had have all gone - skin allergies, stomach problems, persistent respiratory infections, joint pain, tiredness, irritability and anxiety. I still suffer mild asthma which is quickly relieved with the NGC therapy.

I have included dozens of peer-reviewed scientific evidence as well as testimonials from patients, to support the use of the NGC therapy. My patients who have tried NGC therapy have either completely replaced their medications with NGC therapy or have reduced their prescription drugs to a fraction of what it used to be.

I have arranged this book into four main sections. Those in a hurry can jump straight into Section 3 to get started with the therapy. I have also discussed some critical factors that affect the progression of asthma and invariably the outcome of the NGC therapy.

The aim of this book is to show those living with asthma that there is a complimentary or alternative therapy for asthma, which at the very least, will improve their quality of life: for many it will dramatically reduce or eliminate their symptoms. I believe you will find the advice inside this book extremely helpful and possibly life-saving. The NGC therapy has changed my life and the lives of many of my patients for the better, and I sincerely hope it does the same for anyone experiencing asthma.

The Problem with the Current Medical Management of Asthma

Asthma is the result of a dysfunctional immune system causing a hypersensitivity to substances that are harmless to most people. The function of the immune system is to keep track of foreign substances entering the body and to provide protection against such elements which include microorganisms, abnormal proteins, environmental toxins and cancer cells. A properly functioning immune system is intelligent enough to react only to those foreign substances that have the potential to cause harm, saving the body from the enormous stresses that occur when the immune system is activated.

In asthma, the immune system has a flawed recognition system and overreacts to many harmless foreign elements. This abnormal reaction results in the generation of excessive amounts of inflammation-causing chemicals such as histamine, leukotrienes and free radicals.

THE ROLE OF FREE RADICALS IN ASTHMA

Free radicals are the primary cause of severe inflammation responsible for asthma and other chronic diseases such as Diabetes and Alzheimer's. Inflammation is the medical term describing an injury occurring inside the body. When people prone to asthma come in contact with allergens (irritating toxins), their lungs produce massive amounts of free radicals and other chemicals that fuel inflammation. Free radicals are also produced in health during energy generation inside cells, and to counteract the inflammation they cause, the body employs compounds called antioxidants. Antioxidants are crucial for preventing inflammation and damage to hard-working organs of the body such as the lungs and heart. Studies show that low levels of antioxidants in the lungs encourage inflammation and increase the risk of developing chronic diseases such as asthma. (Rahman I, MacNee W, 2000)

Although inflammation precedes every disease, in reality inflammation is the normal response of the body to injuries and foreign contaminants. Inflammation acts as an early warning signal for the body to send out immune cells to repair an injury or contain a toxic compound.

Diseases such as asthma, however, cause a hypersensitivity of the body's immunity resulting in chronic inflammation and eventual weakening of the immune system.

A weak immune system is incapable of defending the body against opportunistic microbes responsible for recurrent chest infections common in asthma.

The resulting inflammatory injury to the airways triggered by allergens and infections produces copious amounts of thick mucus that congest the chest and airways and cause the symptoms seen in asthma.

The cycle of inflammation, dysfunctional immunity, persistent infections and deficiency of essential chemicals are what sustain chronic asthma. Managing these problems requires an entirely different approach to current hospital protocols.

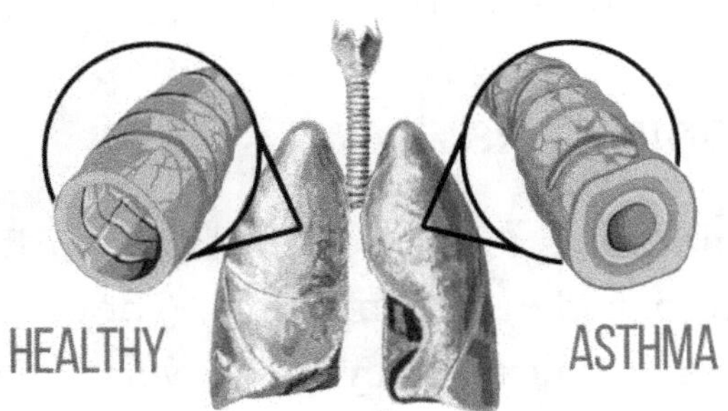

HOW HOSPITALS MANAGE ASTHMA

Hospitals manage asthma mainly by using two drug classes - Bronchodilators (Relievers) and Steroids (Preventers). In place of Bronchodilators, Anticholinergics, a different drug type, are used. Leukotriene modifiers such as Singulair also belong to a different group and are sometimes used in place of steroids. Antibiotics and antihistamines are also frequently prescribed for asthma. Many of the newer drugs prescribed today are a combination of steroids and bronchodilators like Advair which is a combination of fluticasone (steroid) and salmeterol (bronchodilator).

The aim of hospital management of asthma is to keep the airways open with bronchodilators and to prevent inflammation with steroids. While such a management protocol will help alleviate ongoing symptoms of asthma, it fails to address the underlying causes which when left untreated results in worsening symptoms and chronic asthma. Prescription drugs also cause serious side effects from long-term use.

BRONCHODILATORS

Bronchodilators such as Salbutamol (Albuterol in the US) help widen the airways. They are usually available as inhalers; they work very fast and are useful in emergencies. Salbutamol provides a quick but short-lasting relief from asthma. Longer lasting bronchodilators typically contain steroids and include brands like Symbicort and Serevent.

Bronchodilators produce their primary effect on the airways and lungs, however, they also stimulate the heart and cause such side effects as irregular and rapid heartbeat, anxiety and heart damage. Other common side effects of bronchodilators are tiredness, irritability and headaches. Bronchodilators also inhibit absorption of magnesium and cause magnesium deficiency - one of the leading causes of bronchospasms and narrowing of the airways. Clinical studies have demonstrated a link between asthma and low levels of magnesium in the blood. (Landon and Young, 1993).

STEROIDS

Steroids have very powerful anti-inflammatory properties and are used to manage an ever-growing list of diseases including asthma. The symptoms of asthma - Shortness of breath, Wheezing and Coughing, can all be traced to inflammation, and suppressing inflammation will invariably help with these symptoms.

Steroids produce their anti-inflammatory effect by switching off the genes that control inflammation.

Inflammation, however, is crucial and alerts the body to ongoing damage and instigates the healing process.

By interfering with genes, the anti-inflammatory effects of steroids affect the whole body, not just the airways, and over time the natural healing process initiated by inflammation is suppressed, leading to the many side effects typically associated with long-term use of steroids.

These side effects are very common in older people with asthma and include - joint pains, heart disease, persistent skin and chest infections, diabetes and depression.

Long-term use of steroids suppresses the immune system and increases the risk of chest infections, a common problem in asthma. Steroids also destroy natural antioxidants in the body that are vital for controlling inflammation in the lungs. Furthermore, steroids damage the digestive system and cause nutrient deficiencies which are common in asthma and known to contribute to the disease.

ANTICHOLINERGIC DRUGS

Anticholinergic drugs block the neurotransmitter (nerve chemical) acetylcholine which helps relax the airways and widen the breathing tubes. Ipratropium is a commonly prescribed Anticholinergic medication. The common side effects of anticholinergics are dry mouth and eyes, dizziness, abnormal heart rate.

ANTIBIOTICS

The immune system is typically depressed in asthma resulting in frequent chest infections. Inevitably people with asthma are very often prescribed antibiotics which cause further damage to the immune system. (Yusuke Shono et al., 2016).

Antibiotics slow down the activity of immune cells whose function it is to defend the body against harmful bacteria and instead destroy beneficial probiotics that prevent the overgrowth of harmful bacteria such as E. coli and Staphylococcus Aureus. There is scientific evidence linking childhood exposure to antibiotics and asthma. (Kozyrskyj A L et al., 2007).

ANTIHISTAMINES

Antihistamines help relieve the effects of excessive histamine - one of the chemicals produced in asthma and allergies. Histamine encourages the flow of fluid from blood vessels into the airways, causing congestion and narrowing of the breathing tubes. Antihistamines however, interfere with the functions of the brain, nerves and intestines and cause side effects such as drowsiness, memory loss, confusion, nausea and diarrhoea. Recent studies show that prolonged use of antihistamines, as well as anticholinergics, increases the risk of brain diseases including Alzheimer's and Parkinson's diseases. (Shelly L et al., 2015)

Prescription drugs are helpful for controlling the symptoms in asthma, but their long-term use leads to serious complications. Most people with asthma will suffer complications caused by steroids and bronchodilators. The logical conclusion is that prescription medicines for asthma should be best replaced with less toxic alternatives when possible. However, it is extremely dangerous to stop taking asthma medications while trying the NGC therapy. The aim of the therapy is to assist in the gradual withdrawal of prescription medications, if possible. An inhaler should always be within reach while using the treatment and even when symptoms have diminished. Prescription drugs are still the best medications for managing emergency asthma crisis.

The Discovery of NGC Therapy

(Nebulised Glutathione-Colloidal Silver)

When I took an interest in natural medicine after my coma in 2013, I started researching and experimenting with natural remedies. I was mainly interested in trying out substances that naturally occurred in the body and that way the risk of developing side effects will be minimal. Nevertheless, I tried a lot of herbs, extracts, potions and supplements, as well as breathing exercises, salt inhalation and dietary changes, and none provided any satisfactory result. Then I came across information online, suggesting that nebulized glutathione helped with asthma symptoms.

I had come across Glutathione in my research on numerous occasions as a useful supplement for treating cardiovascular diseases and eliminating toxins from organs but had no idea it could help with asthma. I quickly confirmed that only specially prepared Reduced Glutathione was safe for use. I was fascinated by the therapy because I knew enough about Glutathione to realise there was a possibility that it helped. I was also interested in the fact that a nebuliser was used to deliver the drug which indicated a possibility of quick relief with symptoms. Nebulisers deliver drugs more efficiently to the lungs than inhalers and are better for managing lung diseases such as asthma.

I ordered specially prepared L-glutathione and proceeded to try the therapy. Within a few minutes of inhaling the Glutathione, it became apparent that it was different from anything else I had tried previously. I could feel my airways opening and my lungs relaxing and expanding, and I felt my breathing improve.

I was on prescription inhalers and steroid tablets when I started nebulizing Glutathione, and I suffered the tight and heavy chestiness that is familiar to people with asthma, but within minutes I noticed an easing of chest tightness, comparable to the relief from Ventolin inhalers.

Ventolin (Salbutamol) without any doubt is one of the wonder drugs of allopathic medicine. It is probably one of the fastest acting prescription drugs, and on my search for a natural remedy for asthma, I was interested in anything that could provide the same level of relief as Ventolin, and nebulized Glutathione seemed to do exactly that.

As I continued nebulising the glutathione, I noticed that I was producing copious amounts of mucus and had to clear my throat continually. This excessive mucus production continued for many weeks whenever I used the therapy, and as the mucus loosened, my breathing and health improved. In my mind, this excessive and thick mucus is the primary cause of breathing difficulties that occur in asthma.

I nebulized Glutathione until my breathing improved 10 minutes later. I was ecstatic, but my joy started to fade about 2 hours later when I could feel the tightening in my chest returning, a sign for me to reach out for the inhaler.

I used the nebuliser a few more times that day, and the next day I decided to increase the concentration. I had nebulized one capsule (200 mg) of Glutathione in 10mls of water, but this time I doubled the strength and dissolved two (400 mg) in 10mls of water. I felt even better, and the relief lasted for around 6 hours before I felt the need for another session.

I could clearly see that the stronger the glutathione solution, the better the relief achieved. I decided to double the strength again, but this time I used two capsules (400mg) in 5 ml of water, and the result was even better than before, and I went nearly the whole day without needing another session with the nebuliser. I tried increasing the concentration again but realised that very concentrated solutions prevented the nebuliser from functioning properly.

I continued nebulizing glutathione once or twice daily for a few months and observed that my overall health was improving remarkably. My energy levels which had plummeted after the coma were now back up. The chronic joint pain, and abdominal discomfort I also had, completely disappeared. My health continued to get better, and I reduced the nebuliser to just once daily or every other day.

Suddenly, I realised I was using the nebuliser more often, and soon discovered I had developed a chest infection. I was susceptible to chest infections like many people with asthma, and I would take several courses of antibiotics every year. I was aware of the long-term dangers and side effects of antibiotics, particularly with regards asthma, and I avoided them whenever possible.

I decided to treat the chest infection with Colloidal Silver. I was already using Colloidal Silver in my clinic to successfully treat many infectious diseases, having studied scientific literature ascertaining its effectiveness and safety. I decided to nebulise a mixture of Colloidal Silver and Glutathione by dissolving the Glutathione in Colloidal Silver instead of water.

To my amazement, all traces of the chest infection disappeared by the next day. I decided to stay on the mixture, and as the weeks went by, I felt better than I felt on the Glutathione alone. I could feel my lungs expanding more than before, and my energy level was so high I picked up daily cycling as my regular exercise, a sport I continue to this day. It was my first proper exercise in many years. In my opinion, the extra healing benefit I observed with Colloidal Silver is not only because of its powerful antibiotic property, but also because Colloidal Silver accelerates the healing of damaged organs.

As the months went by and I continued nebulising the mixture of Glutathione and Colloidal silver I noticed I stopped having frequent chest infections. Since then, I haven't suffered any more chest infections and the occasional colds I contract only last a few days.

I had been using Colloidal Silver for many months before I realised I had to ascertain that inhaled colloidal silver is as safe as ingesting it. I found several animal studies showing that inhaling over 30 times the amount that I was using, for a longer period, was completely safe. (Jon Ho Ji et al., 2007). Moreover, the body eliminates over 90% of excess silver in the body within a week. It was very clear that the dose of Colloidal Silver I was nebulising was completely safe and too tiny to cause any form of toxicity.

I observed after a while that my need for the nebuliser varied from one month to another. Sometimes I needed it once every few days, and at other times I would use it up to 3 times daily. I only realised after a vacation, that the environment had a greater impact on asthma than I had imagined.

I live in Torrevieja, a booming holiday destination in Spain with a lot of ongoing construction work. I had travelled for the first time since discovering the therapy to Denia, a greener town with far less construction work and cleaner air and I hardly used the nebuliser over there; within a day of returning from the trip, I used the nebuliser several times. I quickly realised that on the days when the air around me seemed relatively clean, for example after rains, I used a lot less of the nebuliser, about once every day or every couple of days, and when the weather turned dusty, I used the nebuliser several times.

I started paying attention to the quality of air around me, and when I acquired an air filter for my home, I noticed I didn't need to use the nebuliser as often even when the air outside was noticeably contaminated.

While I experimented with the NGC (Nebulised Glutathione Colloidal Silver) therapy, I also worked on other aspects of my health. My Health Report from the diagnostic technology I used in my clinic showed I had very high levels of toxins and a decompensated immune system. I also had problems with my digestive and cardiovascular functions. As I worked on my health, first by detoxing my body and then strengthening my immune system, I noticed I didn't need the nebuliser very often, and would go many days without using it. I was correcting the long-term damage of asthma, and every action I took improved my breathing.

I was doing quite well for many months until I realised once again that I required more of the NGC therapy to stay symptom-free. I had hiked through some thick bushes the weekend before and suspected a particularly nasty allergen was responsible. I was too busy to use the nebuliser as often as I needed and didn't want to augment my therapy with an inhaler. Instead, I decided to add about 1 ml of Ventolin Solution to the NGC mix.

As expected, I didn't need to use the nebuliser as often for the next few days, until I was sure the allergy had cleared and reverted to using just the NGC mix. Although the outcome with Ventolin was impressive, I decided not to continue and to use only the NGC solution because Ventolin can cause a form of dependence resulting in 'Lazy Lungs Syndrome'. When Ventolin is used to expand the airways, the muscles that naturally perform this function become weak and cause a reliance on Ventolin. I believe highly inflammatory allergens in the environment are responsible for the occasional extreme symptoms of asthma that many require additional Ventolin.

After two years of using the NGC therapy, I decided to try it on my patients. I had been seeing some patients in my newly established clinic who were aware of the therapy and were keen to start. The first patient was in his early forties when he developed asthma. He was prescribed inhalers and was very concerned about the side effects. He responded very well to the therapy, and after using it for a few months, he reported that he rarely used it except occasionally in the winter months when his symptoms are more severe.

Other patients had equally good outcomes with the therapy, some more so than others. A few with very chronic asthma needed occasional Ventolin.

Nevertheless, everyone who tried the NGC therapy could stop many of their prescription drugs, especially the steroidal inhalers. They had felt greater symptomatic relief with the NGC therapy than with inhalers, and decided to stop some of their prescription medications. They also reported that other health problems had been resolved such as high blood pressure, erectile dysfunction and joint pain.

In my experience, NGC therapy will provide a level of relief for anyone with asthma. However, the extent and depth of healing experienced will depend on the individual's current state of health as well as the level of pollution in their surrounding environment. Improving any of these factors will certainly improve the outcome of NGC therapy.

JENNY KNIGHT

I have suffered from asthma for many years, but the doctors in the UK diagnosed me with bronchitis! It was not until I lived in Mallorca that I was diagnosed with asthma.

This was 17 years ago, and I was given Pulmicort and Terbasmin. I was told to take the Pulmicort every day as a preventative and the Terbasmin as and when necessary. I was also diagnosed with rhinitis and given a nasal spray to take twice a day.

For a while, I was doing ok but every winter I was very poorly. I was given antibiotics and told to have the flu jab every year as I was considered an "at risk" patient.

As time went on these medications did not work so well, and just over three years ago I moved to Torrevieja. A friend of mine told me about Dr Mannu, and I made an appointment to see him. I was pleased and relieved to find someone who could help me. I knew the medications I was taking were steroids and not good for me, but what alternatives were there?

I had the scan at Medb which showed that the steroids were damaging my kidneys, and heart and causing high blood pressure. My immunity was also very low. I knew that asthma had an adverse effect on my immune system, but I didn't know about the rest! I asked him what I could do to alleviate the nasty effects.

Dr Mannu who also suffers asthma, told me that he used himself as a "guinea pig" in trying various natural remedies for asthma and had found an effective treatment consisting of nebulising Glutathione (helps to dissolve and get rid of the "gunk"), Colloidal Silver, and occasional Ventolin.

He let me try this at his clinic especially when I felt poorly, and I felt immediate relief, and so much better afterwards. After a few times, I decided to purchase a kit and start with the therapy. Within a few days, I felt incredible relief from the treatment. Nowadays, I use it about three times daily in the winter months when my asthma is more severely, and not so often in the summer months or not at all for many days.

I am happy to say that since I have been using the nebuliser, I have stopped taking the steroid puffers, over a period, and I feel so much better. In fact, many people have asked me if I have lost weight! I have indeed lost some body fat, and Dr Mannu told me that the Glutathione regulates the body's metabolism and therefore the body is working as it should.

Discovering the NGC therapy is the best thing that happened to me as well as the fact that I can manage my asthma much better on my own without taking horrible steroids.

WHAT IS NGC THERAPY?

NGC Therapy consists of Nebulising Glutathione, Colloidal Silver and Optional Ventolin.

WHAT IS NEBULISATION?

Nebulisation describes the process of using a nebuliser for administering medications. A nebuliser uses compressed air, ultrasonic-frequency or other non-chemical means to break up liquids into aerosol droplets for inhalation. Nebulisers are the most efficient way to deliver drugs to the lungs.

The lungs have one of the richest blood vessel densities in the body, giving them a large surface area for absorbing drugs. Unlike inhalers that use chemical propellants to deliver drugs into the lungs, nebulisers only deliver the pure drug to the lungs. Moreover, in comparison to inhalers, nebulisers produce finer drug particles that travel deeper into the lungs, resulting in a quicker and longer lasting relief from asthma symptoms.

GLUTATHIONE

Glutathione is the most powerful antioxidant in the lungs. The primary function of antioxidants, such as glutathione, is to neutralise toxic chemicals called free radicals that are the underlying cause of asthma and many other chronic diseases. Many studies show that people with asthma are chronically deficient in glutathione. (Kathy T. Schroer et al.,2011; Anne M. Fitzpatrick et al., 2011). The outcome of glutathione deficiency in asthma is that toxic free radicals flood the airways and lungs causing intense inflammation and breathing difficulties.

Free radicals are highly reactive chemicals produced by allergens and toxic chemicals. They are also a by-product of respiration and energy production in the body, and to counteract their harmful effect; the lungs produce glutathione, a powerful antioxidant.

Among the many different antioxidants found in the body, Glutathione is considered the most crucial. It has been described as 'The mother of all antioxidants' because it is essential for recycling other antioxidants in the body including Vitamin C, Vitamin E, CoQ10 and Selenium. Invariably, deficiency of Glutathione results in a deficiency of many other essential antioxidants. Antioxidants such as Glutathione are considered the singular most important group of compounds for preventing chronic diseases, slowing down the ageing process and rejuvenating the body.

Glutathione occurs everywhere in the body but is most abundant in the lungs where its concentration is 140 times that of blood. In the lungs, Glutathione prevents the build-up of toxic free radicals directly responsible for asthma attacks.

Glutathione is also critical for protecting major organs and preventing disease. It is essential for reducing oxidative stress in the brain and helps prevent chronic diseases linked to oxidative stress, such as Parkinson's and Alzheimer's diseases.

The eyes contain very high concentrations of glutathione required to keep the lens transparent, and studies show that glutathione protects the eyes from diseases such as glaucoma, cataracts and retinal damage. Glutathione also facilitates the immune system by protecting young immune cells from damage and enhancing the activities of Natural Killers cells – immune cells responsible for fighting viruses.

Glutathione exists in two forms inside the body - the reduced and oxidised forms. When glutathione is in its reduced form, it is active and ready to neutralise toxic free radicals, however, during the process, reduced glutathione is used up and is transformed into its oxidised or inactive form.

In a healthy person, 90% of Glutathione is in the reduced or active form, and only 10% is in the oxidised or inactive form. The reverse is the case with asthma, where reduced or active glutathione is either depleted or not enough produced in the first place, causing a build-up of free radicals that trigger asthma.

Studies show that people with asthma are genetically predisposed to glutathione deficiency. (Sherif M. Abdel-Alim et al., 2007). The implication is that people affected will have a higher risk of developing asthma when exposed to factors that increase the demand for Glutathione such as foreign proteins and allergens. These foreign proteins trigger the production of enormous quantities of toxic free radicals which are the primary cause of asthma.

VACCINES AND ASTHMA

Studies have demonstrated a link between vaccines and childhood asthma. (Kemp T et al., 1997). Vaccines typically contain many foreign proteins and toxic chemicals including animal proteins, Formaldehyde, Polysorbate 80 and Phenol carbolic acid. These proteins cause intense inflammation in a young human body and cause severe damage and dysfunction, especially to the vulnerable immune system.

At birth and during infancy, the immune system is still immature and requires time to become aware of its environment and determine the most appropriate response to foreign substances. Exposing the body to vaccines early in life can distort the immune system in susceptible people and cause diseases such as asthma.

Children therefore, with a genetic defect that compromises Glutathione production in the body have an increased risk of developing diseases like asthma when exposed to vaccines or other toxic chemicals that promote free radical production and inflammation.

HOW NEBULIZING GLUTATHIONE TACKLES ASTHMA

Nebulizing Glutathione restores depleted Glutathione reserves in the body which helps neutralise the underlying cause of asthma - Free Radicals and provides quick relief from asthma symptoms as well as long-term health benefits. The capacity of Glutathione to neutralise inflammation-causing Free Radicals, make it a potent anti-inflammatory agent in the lungs.

Glutathione is also a powerful mucolytic and breaks down thick mucus blocking breathing tubes. The impact of mucus in asthma became evident to me when I started nebulizing Glutathione and noticed that my breathing improved as mucus cleared from my lungs.

Glutathione increases the volume of air entering the lungs as well as the oxygen saturation of red blood cells resulting in more oxygen carried to the tissues. Studies also show that Glutathione reduces the damage caused by smoking. (Neal S Gould et al., 2015).

HOW GLUTATHIONE HELPS PREVENT COMPLICATIONS

In addition to preventing and treating asthma, Glutathione provides many benefits that prevent health complications common in people with asthma. By tackling the cause of inflammation rather than inflammation itself, Glutathione helps preserve the valuable benefits of inflammation, without causing any side effects, unlike steroids which control inflammation by suppressing genes and cause many side effects. Inflammation is a useful process in the body when controlled, and helps inform the body of injury and initiates healing. However, when excessive, it causes diseases.

The anti-inflammatory properties of glutathione help protect organs from damage and prevent chronic diseases such as heart failure, diabetes, kidney failure, cataracts, weight gain, chronic fatigue and Cancer. (Khalid Rahman, 2007).

Glutathione is also crucial for keeping the immune system healthy which helps prevent recurrent infections common in asthma. (Anne M Fitzpatrick et al., 2011). It is also a powerful detoxification agent essential for removing harmful toxins from the body, especially the lungs and liver.

Glutathione is particularly useful for older people with asthma who nearly always suffer from heart diseases caused by repeated use of bronchodilators and steroids. Long-term use of steroids will eventually lead to high blood pressure and cardiovascular diseases. Bronchodilators such as Ventolin also cause high blood pressure as well as irregular heartbeats.

Glutathione prevents free radical build-up and protects the blood vessels and heart against inflammation and injury. One key benefit of glutathione is that it boosts energy levels.

FOOD SOURCES OF GLUTATHIONE

The best food sources of Glutathione are eggs, milk, meat, asparagus, watermelon, avocado, kale and cauliflower.

THE RECOMMENDED FORM OF GLUTATHIONE

Only the reduced form of Glutathione specially prepared for nebulization is safe to use. Any other Glutathione can cause bronchospasm (tightening of the chest) and breathing problems.

COLLOIDAL SILVER – POWERFUL ANTIBIOTIC AND HEALING AGENT

Colloidal Silver has properties that make it an indispensable ally in preventing and treating asthma. It is a powerful antibiotic capable of destroying viruses, bacteria, fungi and parasites, unlike most prescription antibiotics that are only effective against bacteria. Colloidal Silver produces potent anti-inflammatory and antihistamine effects in the lungs. It also accelerates the healing of damaged airways in asthma.

Silver occurs naturally in the body, and scientists suggest that a silver concentration below .01% of body weight will compromise the immune system and increase the risk of infections. People with asthma have a dysfunctional immune system which makes them prone to chest infections and very often take prescription antibiotics that cause many side effects.

Colloidal Silver is a potent natural antibiotic with no known side-effects, and can effectively take the place of prescription antibiotics for managing infections in asthma.

Silver has been known as a powerful antibiotic for many centuries. The ancient Romans consumed food and water from silverware with the knowledge that silver protected against infectious diseases.

Until the 1930s when chemical antibiotics were introduced and widely promoted, colloidal silver was the drug of choice for fighting infections, and speeding up healing in the body.

Many scientific studies have proven the effectiveness of colloidal silver against viruses, bacteria, fungi and parasites. (See References).

A study in 2005 (Elechiguerra et al.) showed that Colloidal Silver particles stopped HIV from entering cells and infecting the body. Another study published in 2011 (Lara et al.) demonstrated that Colloidal Silver destroyed many viruses and bacteria, including MRSA, HIV-1, Hepatitis virus and ampicillin-resistant E. coli.

Another study from 2013 (Matthew and Kuriakose) found silver particles effective against antibiotic resistant bacteria such as Staph aureus, Pseudomonas and Klebsiella.

Colloidal Silver destroys the respiration and metabolism of bacteria, viruses and fungi by disabling the enzymes that control these processes. Studies also show that silver attaches to the DNA of viruses, stopping them from reproducing and spreading inside cells. Other studies, however, show that colloidal silver may even attach to the surface of viruses and prevent them from entering cells in the first place. Unlike prescription antibiotics, there is no known microbial resistance to Colloidal Silver.

Silver can exist in many different forms, but the best form of silver for therapy is Colloidal Silver. The term 'Colloidal' refers to a solution of suspended particles. The colloidal state is the natural state of fluids inside the body. Blood exists in a colloidal state, and this makes it possible for minerals in their pure and unaltered form to move to different parts of the body.

Colloidal suspensions are the most efficient means of delivering microscopic particles such as silver particles into the body. The strength of Colloidal Silver is calculated in PPM (Parts per million), which is a measure of how many parts of colloidal silver are in a million parts of water. The concentration used for NGC therapy is 20 PPM - 20 parts of Colloidal Silver in 1 million parts of water. At this concentration, colloidal silver is completely harmless.

There are reports of Silver causing a bluish discoloration of the skin called Argyria. This rare condition only happens when people consume the wrong form of silver such as Silver salts. It is unlikely for Argyria to develop even with very high concentrations of Colloidal Silver. According to the World Health Organization (WHO), the body can store up to 10 grammes of Silver without any adverse effects, an impossible concentration to achieve even by consuming several Litres of 20 PPM Colloidal Silver every day for many years. (Ioannis G. Theodorou et al., 2014)

Colloidal Silver must be stored in a dark glass bottle and away from appliances that generate electromagnetic fields such as fridges and computers. Metal containers will also deactivate Colloidal Silver. Colloidal Silver is most active when it is freshly prepared, but it will continue to retain its potency for many years. However, on average it has a shelf-life of about four months.

HOW TO MANAGE ASTHMA WITH NGC (Nebulised Glutathione- Colloidal Silver)

What You Need:

Nebuliser

Colloidal Silver Solution

Reduced Glutathione Capsules

Measuring syringe (5 ml)

Glass container for storage and mixing

ABOUT NEBULISERS

Nebulisers, provide the most efficient route for delivering drugs used to treat lung diseases. Unlike inhalers that require chemicals to propel drugs into the lungs, nebulisers achieve a better result using non-chemical means such as compressed air, ultrasound or vibrating membranes.

The most commonly used nebulisers are called 'Jet nebulisers', and they work by forcing compressed air through liquid medication to create a vapour. Jet nebulisers are cheaper and noisier than the other types. Ultrasonic nebulisers are one of the newer types of nebulisers and are smaller and quieter than Jet nebulisers.

The latest Nebulisers use a vibrating mesh to produce the drug-aerosol. They are silent and small enough to qualify as 'pocket nebulisers'.

Nebulisers have some benefits over inhalers. For a start, nebulisers only require the pure medication to generate the vapour, unlike inhalers that use chemicals to propel drugs into the lungs. In comparison to inhalers, the drug particles produced with nebulisers are finer and travel deeper into the lungs to provide longer lasting relief.

The vapour or mist from nebulisers can be inhaled through the nose using a face mask, or through the mouth with a mouthpiece. Nose inhalation with a face mask is preferable to the mouthpiece as the nose, unlike the mouth, has tiny hairs that can filter out debris. The nebuliser is easy to use and can be managed by children as young as six months old.

The only drawback of nebulisers is that they are cumbersome and are not easy to carry around like inhalers. More compact models referred to as Pocket or Mini nebulisers are quite handy but tend to be slightly more expensive than bulkier types.

HOW TO USE A NEBULISER

Wash your hands and make sure all the parts of the nebuliser are properly connected. There are typically four main parts - the air compressor (nebuliser machine), a plastic tubing, the drug chamber and a mask. Usually, one end of the plastic tubing connects to the air compressor and the other end to the drug chamber which is then attached to a face mask.

The medicine chamber, face mask and tubing, should be disinfected at least once a week. To start using the nebuliser, load the drugs into the drug chamber. Attach the face mask to the drug chamber, secure the face mask to your head with the strap, turn the machine on and then breathe normally.

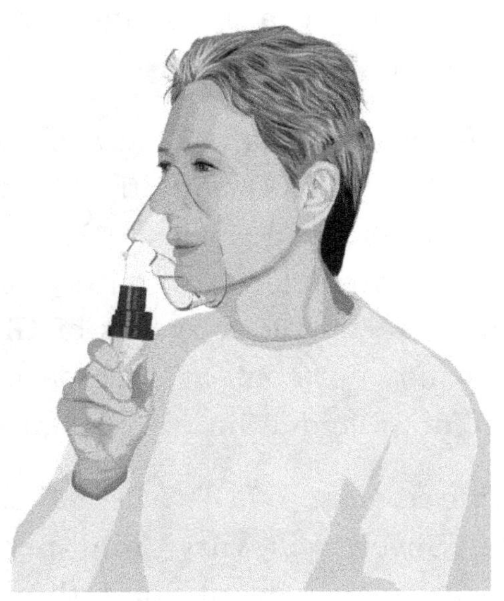

THE NGC THERAPY TECHNIQUE

Empty two capsules of Glutathione (400 mg) into a glass container (eggcup) containing 7.5 ml of 20 ppm Colloidal Silver solution. Glutathione dissolves very quickly with a hissing sound. Add about 2 ml of the mixture into the nebuliser drug holder (Add enough to fill the drug chamber without overloading it). Secure the mask, switch on the nebuliser and then inhale the mist and breathe in normally.

The vapour has a slight smell of Sulphur but feels smooth and painless during inhalation. Use for 5-

15 minutes, as often as required, usually about three times daily. The mixture should be used immediately or within the day, to avoid possible oxidation of the glutathione and a weakening of the NGC solution.

Children younger than 12 years old should take half the dose - 200 mg in 7.5 ml of 20 PPM Colloidal Silver. Sometimes, when the mixture is too concentrated (occurs with some brands of Colloidal Silver or older stocks of Glutathione), the nebuliser may not spin. In such cases, add an extra 1 or 2 ml of Colloidal Silver to the mix.

The required dose of NGC (Nebulised Glutathione Colloidal Silver) will vary from person to person depending on the severity of asthma. While some people will need to use it just once a day to experience significant relief of symptoms, others may need to use it more often to achieve the same relief. Nevertheless, as the lungs heal and symptoms subside, the therapy sessions will reduce.

There is no risk of overdosing with Colloidal Silver or Glutathione. However, to avoid a possible weakening of the Glutathione by Colloidal Silver, it is important to alternate every week or fortnightly between nebulising pure Glutathione and the NGC solution.

NEBULISING GLUTATHIONE ALONE

Nebulized Glutathione on its own is sufficient to improve breathlessness and other symptoms of mild to moderate forms of asthma.

To nebulise glutathione alone, dissolve one or two capsules of glutathione (200 - 400 mg) in 7.5 – 15 ml of pure water and inhale for 10 - 15 minutes as often as required.

NEBULISING COLLOIDAL SILVER ALONE

Colloidal Silver can be nebulised on its own to treat severe chest infections. To nebulise Colloidal Silver, add about 2 ml of 20 PPM Colloidal Silver to the nebuliser and use for 10-15 minutes, one to three times a day for about ten days. Most chest infections will disappear within ten days of nebulising Colloidal Silver. Individuals prone to chest infections can use Colloidal Silver for longer periods, but it is recommended to allow a week of rest every month to allow the body to excrete excessive silver from the body.

NGC - VENTOLIN COMBINATION

Those with very severe asthma may benefit during periods of severe attack by adding about 1 ml of Ventolin Solution to the NGC solution and nebulising for a few days. Ventolin is a bronchodilator and widens the airways which allow more nebulised medications into the lungs and produces a quicker effect.

A very tiny amount of Ventolin is required to alleviate asthma attacks when combined with the NGC solution, and it appears that the NGC Solution enhances the effect of Ventolin. However, it is important to stop using Ventolin as soon as possible to prevent the likelihood of developing ' Ventolin Dependency'.

Ventolin solution is very cheap and comes in small 10 ml bottles sold over the counter. Those that may require a prescription should inform their doctors of their intention to start using a nebuliser, and usually, that will be enough to get a prescription.

WHAT TO EXPECT WHILE NEBULISING

The NGC therapy will ease breathing difficulties within a few minutes of use. As Glutathione dissolves mucus congesting the airways, there may be a need to clear the throat often.

The lungs and the airways expand to let in more air, and many people describe feeling as if they are using parts of the lungs they haven't used in many years.

The NGC therapy produces a progressive healing effect on the airways and lungs, and over time the treatment can be adjusted according to needs, and in time most people require less and less or have no need for it at all.

A key advantage of NGC therapy is that it boosts energy levels, a huge benefit for people with asthma who typically have low energy levels. Glutathione also boosts the immune system which helps reduce chest infections that are common in asthma. (Pietro Ghezi, 2011).

Colloidal Silver is a powerful antibiotic, antihistamine and anti-inflammatory agent and helps speed up the healing of damaged airways.

The aim of NGC therapy is to improve the symptoms and quality of life of people living with asthma and to replace prescription drugs where and when possible.

The NGC therapy will provide immense benefit for anyone using it. While most people will notice a progressive improvement in symptoms, a few will notice that the benefits plateau after a while. When this occurs, it is most likely due to other complicating problems such as persistent allergens in the environment, mineral deficiencies and chronic inflammation.

JIM

I first became aware that I had asthma when I was about 30 years old, I am now 71. I had been very active all my working life and had also played many sports including football. I knew I was beginning to have a 'breathing' problem but thought it was a chest infection and would let it pass. However, I suffered a very severe asthma attack and had to go to the hospital. At the time, they thought I had suffered a heart attack, but tests showed I hadn't, and then I was seen by the asthma consultant and correctly diagnosed.

I was given a Ventolin 'pump', and I attended the asthma clinic for the next six weeks and all was well; however, I was warned that my breathing would very slowly deteriorate with age. I was advised that I would have to be very careful concerning contracting flu, coughs, colds or any chest infection, as my asthma condition would severely worsen the effects of such illnesses.

In 2001, I bought a house in Cabo Roig, Spain and begun to regularly spend some of the winters in Spain, by 2006 my wife and I were spending virtually six months in Spain. I started having problems with my breathing even though I believed I was living in the healthiest part of the world, Alicante in Spain. I was puzzled. On my return to the UK in the May of 2006, I saw my GP and was prescribed the medication 'Becotide' to be used (2 puffs) morning and night, daily as a preventative. I was still using the Ventolin as and when I felt necessary.

I used the Becotide for the next six years but sometimes, particularly when in the UK, I stopped using it sometimes for a few months. I seemed to have to use it while in Spain mainly. By 2012, while still on the Becotide, I realised I was prone to bleeding at the slightest injury. I assumed my blood was getting thinner with age but in every other aspect, weight, diet and fitness, I was particularly healthy. I had queried my GP in the UK but not received any satisfactory explanation, particularly when I asked about how much steroids were in the Becotide. In fact, I was told it was a negligible amount and would have no lasting effect and was not responsible for my 'blood spots'.

About 2012, my wife had health problems which resulted in her visiting Dr Mannu's surgery and having a full scan. During the visit, I discussed my issues with Dr Mannu as he also has asthma. He explained that in fact, the air where I lived in Orihuela Costa Spain, is particularly bad for people with asthma, due to the dust created by ongoing building projects! Dr Mannu also explained that the

Becotide could be responsible for my bleeding problems.

I was keen to find an alternative to the Becotide as I have always been reluctant to take manufactured medicines due to side effects.

Dr Mannu suggested I try his NGC therapy. I was very susceptible to colds and chest infections, and he explained that the Colloidal Silver would help prevent chest infections. In the past, even with the use of the Becotide, a chest infection had often taken much of the winter to clear, and I was also very poorly during the period. Since starting with the NGC therapy, my health has dramatically improved.

I use the nebuliser, before I go to bed, as and when I feel my breathing or chest is becoming congested or restricted. In truth, my asthma nurse in the UK, who I must see every six months does not agree with my actions. I had to agree to have put on my record that I have refused her advice regarding the Becotide and other even more potent solutions.

I feel it is fair to say that thanks to Dr Mannu we have found a way of staying healthy without resorting to drugs prescribed by our GP and the subsequent side effects.

Environmental and Health Factors Affecting Asthma

DUST

Environmental toxins are the primary trigger of asthma, and the problematic toxin will differ from one person to another. Nevertheless, Dust is a common trigger in many people with asthma.

Dust is far from being the harmless substance many people believe it is and it contains many toxic particles that can cause intense inflammation. In addition to containing inert substances such as carpet fibres, animal hair and plant materials, dust also contains very toxic and harmful substances including lead, pesticides, PCBs (Polychlorinated Biphenyls), mould spores, viruses, bacteria, construction particles and many other toxic organic and chemical substances. Dust from construction sites is particularly toxic and will cause persistent asthma attacks.

Today dust particles are more toxic than they have ever been, and are more likely to trigger allergic reactions that lead to asthma. People living with asthma should avoid dust at all cost. An Air filter is useful for reducing allergens and contaminants in homes and makes a noticeable difference in the quality of health for those with severe asthma. Good Air filters have a dual air filter and ioniser system, with the ioniser helping to settle dust to the ground.

DAMPNESS

Damp buildings are a source of allergens such as bacteria and mycotoxins that trigger asthma or worsen ongoing asthma symptoms. Mycotoxins are highly inflammatory toxins produced by fungi, and many studies link them to severe allergies and lung inflammation. A dehumidifier will be beneficial in buildings or homes with high humidity.

CHLORINE

Chlorinated swimming pools are also a recognised trigger for asthma. Chlorine reacts with water to produce chlorine oxide which studies show cause inflammation of the breathing tubes and lungs.

PETS

Pets are great companions, and there is scientific evidence showing that Pets reduce emotional tension which can be helpful in asthma. However, pet hair is a known trigger of allergic diseases such as asthma.

My first close experience with a pet was with a Cat that adopted me when I relocated to Spain from England. Kibbles was quite charming, and I kept him even though I suspected I might have an allergy to cat hair.

I had him for five years and didn't have problems with him. I would later realise this was because he was very independent and spent most of his time outside and I didn't have to handle cat litter. I adopted a kitten after I lost him, and within weeks, I developed a severe asthma attack that was clearly caused by cat litter. As soon as the kitten was re-homed, the attack very quickly disappeared. In my opinion, the reasons for the acute attack was the cat litter, rather than cat hair.

Nevertheless, in my opinion, people with asthma should avoid pets, especially cats, since cat hair cause more severe irritation of the airways than dog hair. If Pets are unavoidable, they should be discouraged from entering the bedroom.

HOUSEHOLD CHEMICALS AND COSMETICS

Household chemicals and cosmetics are leading sources of toxic substances that trigger asthma, including toothpaste, shower gels, shampoos, shaving creams, deodorants, face creams, body lotions and beauty products of all sorts.

Fabric conditioners contain many toxic chemicals that linger on clothing and slowly exacerbate asthma. Chemical fumes of any type, even when appearing harmless such as air fresheners, are potential asthma triggers.

Alternative products made from non-toxic natural sources should are safer than chemical-based products.

REPLENISH MAGNESIUM

Magnesium is responsible for relaxing the airways and helps prevent narrowing and spasms of the breathing tubes and airways. Magnesium relaxes the entire body which also helps prevent stress induced asthma.

Magnesium deficiency is common in people with asthma, a consequence of long-term use of asthma medications – salbutamol and steroids, that deplete magnesium stored in the body. Studies show that a lack of magnesium in the diet results in reduced

silkworm. The silkworm cocoon secretes serrapeptase to dissolve its casing before emerging as a butterfly. Clinical studies by the discoverer of Serrapeptase, Dr Nieper, as well as studies by many other scientists have demonstrated the capacity of Serrapeptase to dissolve unwanted substances in organs such as plaque in arteries and mucus in the airways, without harming healthy tissue. (A Mazzone et al., 1990).

Serrapeptase also has beneficial anti-inflammatory properties. Serrapeptase will be helpful to people with asthma who still feel heavy congestion with mucus after using the NGC therapy for a few months. Serrapeptase is a relatively cheap supplement, and the recommended dose is 1 – 2 Capsules (90,000 IU per capsule), three times daily for a few weeks or months or until the chest feels less congested.

STRENGTHEN THE LUNGS AND REDUCE ALLERGIES WITH MSM

MSM (Methyl Sulphonyl Methane) is a vital nutrient for producing Collagen, the primary component of the supporting tissues of the body such as the lungs, bones, joints, ligaments, tendons and skin. The consequence of a deficiency in MSM is that people susceptible to lung diseases will develop conditions such as asthma, due to weaknesses in the framework of the lungs.

MSM is essential for building and maintaining the membranes that line the airways which help prevent the allergies that are common in asthma. MSM also helps eliminate toxins in the lungs that fuel inflammation.

MSM regenerates the joints, bones, ligaments, tendons and other structures of the body, in addition to being a powerful painkiller and anti-inflammatory agent which makes MSM a useful supplement for people with long-term asthma who typically suffer from joint and bone diseases.

MSM powder is the best form of MSM and is preferable to tablets and capsules that contain far smaller quantities of MSM as well as being relatively more expensive. A dose of 1 - 2 teaspoons daily will help prevent allergies for those consistently exposed to allergens such as pollen grains in the summer season.

People suffering a severe allergy to pollen grains or other allergic diseases such as eczema should take a full course of MSM for a few months (1 -2 teaspoons in a glass of water, three times daily), before cutting down to a maintenance dose of 1 teaspoon daily.

I suffered severe allergies to pollen grains as well as skin allergies for many years, and both conditions finally disappeared when I started using MSM powder. Today I occasionally take MSM especially if I experience increased sensitivity to pollen or a returning skin lesion. In my opinion, most allergy problems in asthma are caused or worsened by MSM deficiency.

PYCNOGENOL - A RELIABLE ANTI-INFLAMMATORY

Pycnogenol is an extract of French Pine Bark with many healing properties including significant anti-inflammatory benefits. (A Mazzone et al., 1990)

Asthma encourages the production of toxic chemicals responsible for severe and chronic inflammation, and the numerous health benefits of Pycnogenol make it very useful for managing chronic asthma and providing excellent relief. Pycnogenol is an antioxidant and helps neutralise toxic free radicals responsible for the persistent inflammation seen in asthma.

Studies show that Pycnogenol reduces inflammation by switching off the master control switch that regulates inflammation called NF-Kappa B (Nuclear Factor Kappa B). (Raffaella Canali et al., 2009).

Unlike steroids that completely block inflammation - a necessary and useful process in the body,

Pycnogenol reduces inflammation by about 15%, which helps preserve useful inflammatory reactions in the body. On its own, Pycnogenol will provide adequate relief from asthma; however, it does not act quickly and may require up to 6 weeks for the benefits to kick in. It is also expensive in relation to the high dose needed to manage asthma. Pycnogenol will provide relief for people suffering severe and chronic asthma. The required dose for managing asthma symptoms is around 300 mg taken twice daily for a few weeks.

BOOSTING THE IMMUNE SYSTEM WITH VITAMIN D

The hypersensitivity to allergens seen in asthma occurs because of a dysfunctional immune system. It causes further weakening of the immune system, which increases the risk of developing allergies and infections.

Steroid medications prescribed for preventing asthma also depress the immune system and cause other complications that worsen asthma symptoms in time. Vitamin D is an important nutrient for maintaining a healthy immune system and studies show that people suffering asthma are deficient in Vitamin D. (John M Brehm et al., 2010).

Vitamin D is crucial for activating immune cells called T-cells which help the body fight viruses.

Vitamin D is best taken as liquid Vitamin D3 which makes it easier to take the required dose. Although the RDA (Recommended Dietary Allowance) for vitamin D is around 1000 IU daily, studies show that the body can make up to 22,000 IU when exposed to 45 minutes of summer sunlight. A dose of 10,000IU of Vitamin D daily is ideal during the winter months.

Other supplements useful for boosting the immune system are Reishi and Colostrum. Colostrum and Reishi contain several beneficial healing proteins that encourage a strong immunity, including immunoglobulins, Beta Glucans, Peroxidases, Lysozymes, Interferons and many other compounds that are also beneficial for other aspects of health.

ELIMINATE TOXINS FROM THE BODY

Glutathione is a necessary nutrient for the detoxification processes that occur in the lungs and deficiency of Glutathione in asthma will result in higher than normal levels of environmental toxins in the body such as lead, mycotoxins and pesticides.

Glutathione plays a significant role in neutralising harmful free radicals responsible for chronic inflammation and asthma.

The Glutathione in NGC therapy will be sufficient to eliminate toxins in most people with asthma. However, some individuals may require extra help with more powerful detox agents such as Pectasol (Modified Citrus Pectin). Pectasol is an effective oral detox agent backed by numerous scientific studies. It removes toxic substances from the body like lead, mercury, pesticides, mycotoxins, etc. Pectasol is available as capsules and powders.

YOUR DIET IS IMPORTANT

Many studies have linked asthma to nutrient deficiencies. The drugs used primarily for managing asthma - bronchodilators and steroids are known to interfere with nutrient absorption and cause nutrient deficiencies.

People with asthma also have a higher chance of suffering digestive problems which also adds to the problem of nutrient deficiencies. A healthy diet composed of fresh, natural foods is an important aspect of asthma therapy. Food sensitivities tend to be common in asthma, and keeping a record of the diet around the time of an attack may help detect the possible food triggers. Taking a good multivitamin a few times in a year is also a good way of avoiding mineral deficiencies.

FOODS TO AVOID

People with asthma must avoid dairy produce. Milk, cheese and other dairy foods contain abnormal proteins - Casein and Whey proteins that stimulate mucus production in the airways. These proteins also promote excessive secretion of histamine responsible for constricting the airways.

While people with asthma may not be intolerant to lactose in milk, other proteins in milk may cause excessive secretion of mucus from the airways. Dairy produce is also likely to contain toxic proteins from antibiotics and hormones injected into cows to boost milk production.

Goat and sheep's milk are preferable to cow's milk since they contain far less of the irritating proteins seen in Cows products. Soy milk is not a suitable alternative because it contains goitrogens which stop iodine absorption and cause Hypothyroidism (Low thyroid hormones in the body). Soy also prevents absorption of other nutrients and can cause nutrient deficiencies. Almond milk and coconut milk are good alternatives.

Processed foods contain chemicals that modify, enhance and preserve food and are notorious for causing or worsening asthma symptoms. The most worrisome food additives for asthma are Sulphur Dioxide, Sulphites (E221 to 224), Monosodium

Glutamate or MSG (E621 to 623) and Yellow food dye - Tartrazine (E 102). MSG goes by a variety of names on food labels including Hydrolysed vegetable protein, Vegetable or Thai seasoning or Natural flavouring.

All food additives have the potential to trigger asthma symptoms and are potentially dangerous and best avoided. Hydrogenated fats, especially margarine, has been shown by research to increase allergies and asthma in children.

I cut out milk from my diet for many years and felt better for it. Years later, I read that sheep and goat products cause fewer problems, and when I tried sheep cheese and goat's yoghurt, for a while I didn't notice any problems with excessive mucus. Nevertheless, I'll advise people trying the NGC therapy to cut out dairy completely for at least six months, until they are completely free of asthma or feel improved before introducing any form of dairy back into their diet.

HOW EMOTIONS AFFECT ASTHMA

Emotions have a powerful effect on asthma. Negative emotions such as anger, worry and anxiety, are triggers of asthma and contribute to ongoing asthma attacks. Although emotions may worsen asthma attacks, there is no evidence that negative or suppressed emotions cause asthma.

The act of breathing is a primary impulse of life, and anything that hinders this process will create enormous stress in the body. While we can go for days or weeks without water and food, we will all die within minutes without air. People with asthma are constantly hanging on to life for this reason, and this creates an enormous feeling of insecurity. This sense of insecurity worsens just around or before an attack, and the ensuing panic and anxiety will cause hyperventilation and contribute to a worsening of symptoms.

Poor breathing techniques which are common in asthma may also cause a build-up of CO2 that also leads to anxiety. Breathing exercises such as Buteyko Breathing Technique may help retrain the lungs to breathe properly.

But contrary to popular belief, poor breathing is not likely to be a cause of asthma. The fact that people with asthma can go for many weeks or months without any breathing difficulties or even outgrow the illness makes poor breathing an unlikely cause of asthma.

HOW NGC THERAPY WILL HELP WITH ASTHMA COMPLICATIONS

Older people living with asthma will have health problems resulting from long-term use of asthma medications, especially steroids. Some of the most common health problems seen in older asthma sufferers, are also complications of long term steroid use and include joint pain, high blood pressure, heart diseases and diabetes.

NGC therapy reduces or eliminates the need for steroids which helps minimise complications. Glutathione reduces inflammation and helps reduce blood pressure and stabilise blood sugar levels.

Joint pains respond well to MSM which is also very helpful for reducing allergies and strengthening the lungs in asthma. MSM is the main constituent of collagen - the protein that supports bones, joints, skin and the internal framework of the lungs.

Serrapeptase is a useful supplement for dissolving excess mucus in the lungs as well as the plaque in arteries which in turn helps prevent high blood pressure.

EXERCISES

Chronic asthma contracts the lungs and reduces the volume of the lungs and the amount of air entering the airways. Exercises help expand the lungs. Any activity that encourages deep breathing such as cardio exercises will be very helpful.

Swimming is an excellent exercise for asthma. However, the chlorine in chlorinated pools can cause asthma. It is important to avoid pushing the body to the limit during exercises and to allow the body time to rest.

From personal experience, when I skip exercises for a couple of weeks, I notice a tightening of my chest and the need to use NGC more often. For this reason, I exercise at least three times a week. I find vigorous exercises that last a few minutes more helpful than sustained exercises lasting many minutes.

YOU STILL NEED PRESCRIPTION DRUGS

The medications used in hospitals for asthma are undoubtedly life-saving drugs, but they also cause life-threatening long-term complications that reduce the quality of life of people taking them.

It is important for people using the NGC therapy to continue with their prescription drugs and then gradually reduce the dose with the aim of stopping them if possible, however, it is important to have the emergency inhalers handy while trying out the therapy. Prescription inhalers act very quickly and are useful for asthma emergencies.

TRAVELLING

A pocket nebuliser is available and is handy when travelling. Prescription drugs are also necessary while travelling.

THE COST OF THERAPY

Fortunately, the NGC treatment is affordable. The cost of the treatment will reduce in time as the body starts to heal and the amount of medication required reduces. There are many brands of nebulisers available at different prices.

The Omron NE-C28P sells for less than 60 Euros in Amazon and is a very reliable brand. A bottle of Premium Quality Colloidal Solution (100mls) is around 35 Euros and will last for several months. Reduced Glutathione Capsules (120 capsules, 200mg) cost around 60 Euros and should last for up to a year.

WHERE TO GET SUPPLIES

You will find all you need for the therapy from Amazon or online health shops. However, it is important that you get the right quality products. The only form of Glutathione safe for nebulising is Reduced Glutathione specially prepared for nebulisation.

My intention is to make the products available to people with asthma at a cheaper price than anywhere else. You will find the products for NGC therapy from my website:
www.medb.es/wecanbreatheagain.

The only Reduced glutathione I have tried for asthma is L- Glutathione from the company Thera Naturals (www. theranaturals.com). I am very grateful to Michael, the owner of the company for manufacturing such a fantastic and life-saving product.

Get the book from:
http://www.wecanbreatheagain.com.

References

Glutathione

Sherif M. Abdel-Alim, Manal M. El-Masry et al., 2007
Association of Glutathione-S-transferase P1 genotypes with susceptibility to bronchial asthma in children.
Arch Med Sci; 3, 3: 200-207

Comhair SA, Erzurum SC, 2010
Redox control of asthma: molecular mechanisms and therapeutic opportunities.
Antioxid Redox Signal. Jan; 12(1):93-124.

Anne M. Fitzpatrick et al.,2011
Glutathione Oxidation is associated with airway macrophage functional impairment in children with severe asthma.
Pediatr Res. 2011 Feb; 69(2): 154–159.

Kathy T. Schroer et al.,2011
Down-regulation of glutathione S-transferase Pi in
asthma contributes to enhanced oxidative stress.
J Allergy Clin Immunol. 2011 Sep; 128(3): 539–548.

Carroll WD1, Lenney W et al., 2005
Effects of glutathione S-transferase M1, T1 and P1
on lung function in asthmatic families.
Clin Exp Allergy. 2005 Sep;35(9):1155-61.

N. L. A. Misso, K. Powers et al., 1996
Reduced platelet glutathione peroxidase activity
and serum selenium concentration in atopic
asthmatic patients.
Clin Exp Allergy 1996, 26(7):838-847

Y.-L. Lee, Y.-C. Lin et al., 2004
Glutathione S-transferase P1 gene polymorphism
and air pollution as interactive risk factors for
childhood asthma.
Clin Exp Allergy 2004; 34: 1707 - 13

Jonathan Pousky, 2008
The treatment of pulmonary diseases and
respiratory-related conditions with inhaled
nebulized or aerosolized glutathione.
Evid Based Complement Alternat Med. 2008 Mar;
5(1): 27–35.

Rahman I, MacNee W, 2000
Oxidative stress and regulation of glutathione in lung inflammation.
Eur Respir J. 2000 Sep;16(3):534-54.

Fryer AA1, Bianco A, 2000
Polymorphism at the glutathione S-transferase GSTP1 locus. A new marker for bronchial hyperresponsiveness and asthma.
Am J Respir Crit Care Med. 2000 May;161(5):1437-42.

Wisnewski AV, Liu Q, Liu J, Redlich CA, 2005
Glutathione protects human airway proteins and epithelial cells from isocyanates.
Clin Exp Allergy. 2005 Mar;35(3):352-7.

Neal S Gould et al., 2015
Glutathione depletion accelerates cigarette smoke-induced inflammation and airspace enlargement.
Toxicol Sci. 2015 147(2): 466 - 478

Khalid Rahman, 2007
Studies on free radicals, antioxidants and cofactors.
Clinical Interv ageing. 2007 Jun; 2(2): 219 – 236

Pietro Ghezi, 2011
Role of glutathione in immunity and inflammation in the lung.
Int J Gen Med. 2011; 4: 105–113.

COLLOIDAL SILVER

Shahverdi AR1, Fakhimi A et al., 2007
Synthesis and effect of silver nanoparticles on the antibacterial activity of different antibiotics against Staphylococcus aureus and Escherichia coli.
Nanomedicine. 2007 Jun; 3(2):168-71

Panacek A, Kvítek L et al., 2006
Silver colloid nanoparticles: synthesis, characterization, and their antibacterial activity.
J Phys Chem B. 2006 Aug 24;110(33):16248-53

Guzman M, Dille J, Godet S, 2011
Synthesis and antibacterial activity of silver nanoparticles against gram-positive and gram-negative bacteria.
Nanomedicine. 2011 Jun 2.

Khan SS, Mukherjee A, Chandrasekaran N, 2011
Studies on the interaction of colloidal silver
nanoparticles (SNPs) with five different bacterial
species.
Colloids Surf B Biointerfaces. 2011 Oct
1;87(1):129-38.

T. J. Berger, J. A. Spadaro et al., 1976
Effects of electrically generated silver Ions:
Quantitative effects on bacterial and mammalian
cells.
Antimicrob Agents Chemother. 1976 Feb; 9(2):
357–358.

Lu Li, Sun RW et al., 2008
Silver nanoparticles inhibit hepatitis B virus
replication.
Antivir Ther. 2008;13(2):253-62.

N. E. Bogdanchikova, A. V. Kurbatov et al., 2004
Activity of Colloidal silver preparations towards
smallpox virus.
Pharmaceutical Chemistry Journal 2004 December

D. Acharya, P. Pandey et al., 2016
Optical properties of synthesised Colloidal Silver nanoparticles and their antibacterial effects.
Journal of Bionanosci, Vol 10, No 6, Dec 2016, pp. 511-515(5)

Humberto H Lara, Elsa N Garza-Treviño et al., 2011
Silver nanoparticles are broad-spectrum bactericidal and virucidal compounds.
Journal of Nanobiotechnology 2011 9:30

Jose Luis Elechiguerra, Justin L Burt et al., 2005
Interaction of silver nanoparticles with HIV-1.
Journal of Nanobiotechnology 2005 3:6

Mathew TV, Kuriakose S, 2013
Studies on the antimicrobial properties of colloidal silver nanoparticles stabilised by bovine serum albumin.
Colloids Surf B Biointerfaces. 2013 Jan 1; 101:14-8

Berger TJ, Spadaro JA et al., 1976
Antifungal properties of electrically generated metallic ions.
Antimicrob Agents Chemother. 1976 Nov;10(5):856-60.

Woo Kyung Jung, Hye Cheong Koo et al., 2008
Antibacterial Activity and Mechanism of Action of
the Silver Ion in Staphylococcus aureus and
Escherichia coli.
Appl Environ Microbiol. 2008 Apr; 74(7): 2171–
2178.

Pokrowiecki R, Zareba T et al., 2013
Evaluation of biocidal properties of silver
nanoparticles against cariogenic bacteria.
Med Dosw Mikrobiol. 2013;65(3):197-206.

Wright JB, Lam K et al., 1999
Efficacy of topical silver against fungal burn wound
pathogens.
Am J Infect Control. 1999 Aug;27(4):344-50.

Deitch EA, Marino AA et al., 1987
Silver nylon cloth: in vitro and in vivo evaluation of
antimicrobial activity.
J Trauma. 1987 Mar;27(3):301-4.

Ioannis G. Theodorou et al., 2014
Inhalation of Silver Nanomaterials—Seeing the
Risks.
Int J Mol Sci. 2014 Dec; 15(12): 23936–23974

S Takenaka et al., 2001
Pulmonary and systemic distribution of inhaled ultrafine silver particles in rats.
Environ Health Perspec. 2001 Aug; 109(Suppl 4):547 - 551

Amara L Holder et al., 2013
Toxicity of Silver Nanoparticles at the Air-Liquid Interface.
BioMed Research Inter Vol 2013, Article ID 328934

Jae Hyuck Sung et al., 2011
Acute Inhalation Toxicity of Silver Nanoparticles.
Toxicology and Industrial Health 2011, 27 (2): 149-54

Jon Ho Ji et al., 2007
28 Day inhalation toxicity study of Silver nanoparticles in Sprague-Dawley Rats.
Inhal Toxicol 2007 Aug;19(10):857-71

ASTHMA

Current Allergy and Asthma Reports
The role of lung inflation in airway hyperresponsiveness and asthma.
March 2004, Volume 4, Issue 2, pp 166–174

Landon R. A, Young E.A, 1993
The role of magnesium in the regulation of lung function.
J Am Diet Assoc. 1993 Jun;93(6):674-7.

Pulm Med. 2016; 2016:1643717.
Serum Magnesium and Vitamin D Levels as Indicators of Asthma Severity.
Shaikh M.N, Malapati B.R et al., 2016

Kemp T et al
Is infant immunisation a risk factor for childhood asthma or allergy?
Epidemiology. 1997 Nov;8(6):678-80.

Kozyrskyj A L et al., 2007
Increased risk of childhood asthma from antibiotic use in early life.
Chest. 2007 Jun;131(6):1753-9.

Bjerg A et al., 2015
Gas, dust, and fumes exposure is associated with mite sensitization and with asthma in mite-sensitized adults.
Allergy, Volume 70, Number 5, 1 May 2015, pp. 604-607

Wang J et al., 2009
Effect of environmental allergen sensitization on
asthma morbidity in inner-city asthmatic children.
Cli & Exper Allergy, Vol 39, No 9, September 2009,
pp. 1381-1389(9)

Reuser T et al., 1992
Acute angle closure glaucoma occurring after
nebulized bronchodilator treatment with
ipratropium bromide and salbutamol.
J R Soc Med. 1992 Aug; 85(8): 499–500.

Raffaella Canali et al., 2009
The anti-inflammatory pharmacology of Pycnogenol
in humans involves COX-2 and 5-LOX mRNA
expression in leukocytes.
Int Immunopharm Vol 9, Issue 10, Set 2009, Pages
1145 - 1149

A Mazzone et al., 1990
A review of the French maritime pine bark extract
Pycnogenol a herbal medication with a diverse
clinical pharmacology.
Int J Clin Pharmacol Ther. 2002 Apr;40(4):158-68.

A Mazzone et al., 1990
Evaluation of Serratia Peptidase in Acute or
Chronic Inflammation of Otorhinolaryngology
Pathology: A Multicentre, Double-Blind,
Randomised Trial versus Placebo.
Journal of Int Med Research. Sept 1990

Sedighi M, et al., 2006
Low magnesium concentration in erythrocytes of
children with acute asthma.
Iran J Allergy Asthma Immunol. 2006

Shaikh MN, et al., 2016
Serum Magnesium and Vitamin D Levels as
Indicators of Asthma.
Pulm Med. 2016

John M Brehm et al., 2010
Serum vitamin D levels and severe asthma
exacerbations in the Childhood Asthma
Management Program study.
Jor of Allergy and cli immu Volume 126, Issue 1,
July 2010, Pages 52–58. e5

Yusuke Shono et al., 2016
Increased GVHD-related mortality with broad-spectrum antibiotic use after allogeneic hematopoietic stem cell transplantation in human patients and mice.
Sci Trans Med. 18 May 2016, Vol. 8, Issue 339, pp. 339ra71

Shelly L et al., 2015
Cumulative Use of Strong Anticholinergics and Incident Dementia.
JAMA Internal Medicine, 2015;
DOI:10.1001/jamainternmed.2014.7663

About the Author

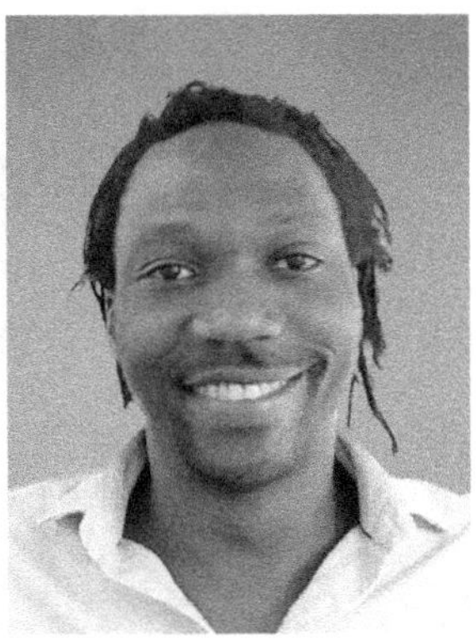

Dr Machi Mannu

Dr Mannu is a writer, researcher and medical doctor practising natural medicine. He has a keen interest in Diagnostic Medicine and manages MedB Diagnostic Centre, a diagnostic and natural healing centre in Alicante, Spain. Since 2012 he has investigated natural therapies supported by scientific studies, and continues to compile a list of the most effective natural remedies. To get in touch with Dr Mannu visit his website: **wwww.medb.es**

It has been a pleasure and an education to have been a patient of Dr Mannu for over three years. I have benefited from his professionalism and expertise. His monthly magazine is full of information, clearly expressed and I Have eagerly looked forward to the publication of his new book.

D H Alexander

www.ingramcontent.com/pod-product-compliance
Lightning Source LLC
Chambersburg PA
CBHW051654060726

47593CB00021B/1083